Move Your Body

JOURNAL TO ELEVATE YOUR LIFE

Using a journal is simply writing down your thoughts and feelings to understand them more clearly. And if you struggle with stress, depression, or anxiety, keeping a journal can help you gain control of your emotions and improve your mental health as well as your your physical health.

ISBN-13: 978-1724833488
ISBN-10: 1724833480

The reason I
exercise today is
for the quality of
life I enjoy.
~ Kenneth H. Cooper

Great things come
to those who sweat
it out!

Every journey
begins with a
single step.

Don't find time to
exercise...
Make time to
exercise!

Exercise is a celebration for what your body can do. It's not a punishment for what you ate!

Love yourself
enough today to
exercise!

Remember that any exercise is better than no exercise!

Fitness is not about being better than someone else....
It is about being better than you used to be!

Exercise is a journey, not a destination.
It must be continued for the rest of your life.
~ Kenneth H. Cooper

Exercise should be regarded as tribute to the heart.

~ Gene Tunney

In 2 weeks you'll
feel it.
In 4 weeks you'll
see it.
In 8 weeks you'll
hear it!

The only bad
workout is the one
you didn't do!

9 781724 833488